DEEP SLEEP

*Unlocking the Secrets to Restorative
and Rejuvenating Sleep
(2023 Guide for Beginners)*

Lulu Fowler

Contents

Chapter 1: Understanding Deep Sleep Hypnosis

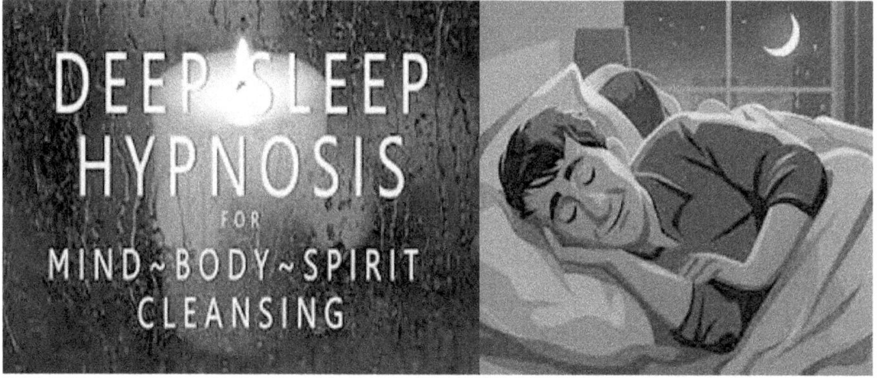

Deep Sleep Hypnosis refers to a technique where a hypnotherapist guides individuals through the power of suggestion to induce sleep. Hypnotherapists employ various methods such as attention, relaxation, and imagery to facilitate symptom management. By using phrases like "relax," "profound," "pure," and "let go," the hypnotist aims to encourage a person to enter a state of deep sleep.

Some people use sleep hypnosis as a tool to aid their sleep. It involves guided thoughts that help direct a person's mind, making it easier for them to fall asleep. While there are many sleep hypnosis options available for download on computers or phones, it remains uncertain whether they are effective. If you are considering sleep hypnosis, continue reading to learn more about it and discover alternative approaches to improve your sleep.

Does Sleep Hypnosis Work?

The effectiveness of hypnotherapy may vary from person to person depending on their level of suggestibility, which refers to how receptive they are to the practice. Studies have shown that about a quarter of individuals cannot be hypnotized. Additionally, incorporating sleep hypnosis into a comprehensive treatment plan may be necessary to experience any benefits. While hypnosis can be helpful for sleep issues, it may not always be the most successful solution.

What Can You Try Instead?

If you are seeking alternative methods to improve your sleep, consider cognitive-behavioral therapy (CBT), which involves examining your sleep habits and working on changing negative thought patterns and anxieties related to sleep. Relaxation techniques such as deep breathing exercises, meditation, and progressive muscle relaxation can also be beneficial. Listening to calming music before bed can help you fall asleep faster and maintain a restful night's sleep.

Although sleep hypnosis is generally considered safe and may offer benefits as an adjunctive sleep aid, there are other effective strategies to explore. It is advisable to consult with your doctor to determine what approach will be most beneficial for you.

Using Self Hypnosis to Achieve Restful Sleep

There can be various reasons why you struggle to sleep at night, ranging from psychological to physical factors. Your sleep environment may not be conducive to a good night's rest, or you may have lingering worries, tasks, or anticipation for the next day keeping you awake. Many of these challenges can be overcome through the practice of self-hypnosis.

Assuming you have already tried conventional remedies and ruled out any underlying health issues, here are some steps you can take to prepare your sleeping environment:

- Create a silent atmosphere by turning off the radio, television, and computer in the background. Silence your mobile phone and try to ensure the rest of the house is quiet.
- Set the temperature to a comfortable level.
- Wear comfortable clothing and have clean sheets on your bed.
- Clear your sleeping area of any clutter, such as crumbs, toys, or other distractions.
- Turn off the lights.
- Before you begin the self-hypnosis process, find a comfortable position that allows you to relax. Take a few deep, slow breaths to initiate the relaxation process.

The self-hypnosis procedure involves visualizing yourself in a warm shower while water fills the bathtub. In your mind, imagine your body gradually relaxing as the water level rises. As the water moves up, envision it soothing and calming your muscles and nerves. Picture your body becoming increasingly relaxed with each upward movement, almost as if the rising water is gently numbing certain areas. During this process, try to keep your body as still as possible and focus on the sensations of relaxation. If any external thoughts or distractions arise, slow down and redirect your attention back to your body.

Ideally, this visualization exercise should help induce a state of deep relaxation, making it easier for you to fall asleep

Chapter 2: The Effects of Deep Sleep on Brain Activity

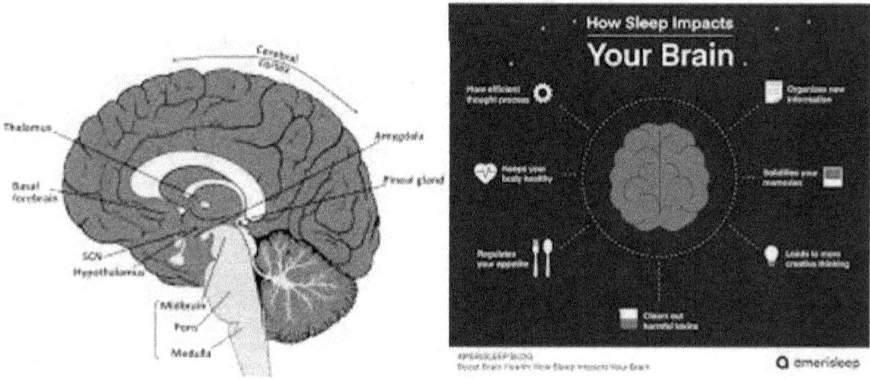

New research using brain imaging techniques has revealed three significant changes in the brain during a hypnotic trance. This chapter explores the findings and their implications.

During a hypnotic trance, as your breathing slows and your body relaxes, your brain activity also undergoes transformations. In a study conducted in the United States, the brains of 57 individuals were monitored during guided hypnosis, and remarkable changes in brain activity and connectivity were observed in certain areas associated with cognitive processes.

The study's results, published in the journal Cerebral Cortex, could potentially enhance the effectiveness of hypnosis in clinical settings, particularly in managing conditions such as pain and post-traumatic stress disorder. Contrary to the stereotypical portrayal of hypnosis with swinging pocket watches and clucking like a chicken, it is increasingly recognized as a scientifically grounded therapeutic approach for various issues, including phobias, trauma, and pain relief.

Typically, a hypnosis session begins with the patient and therapist discussing the desired outcomes. The patient is then guided into a state of deep relaxation and focused attention, during which the therapist reinforces the goals through verbal suggestions and imagery. In highly hypnotizable individuals, these sessions have shown promising results in reducing chronic pain and aiding in smoking cessation. However, the exact mechanisms underlying the hypnotic state and its effects on the brain have remained unclear.

To unravel the mysteries of hypnosis, researchers at Stanford University, led by senior author David Spiegel and lead author Heidi Jiang, conducted a study involving 545 healthy participants. Based on their hypnotizability scores, 38 highly hypnotizable individuals and 21 with low scores were selected. The participants' brain activity was then measured using functional magnetic resonance imaging (fMRI), a technique that detects changes in blood flow within the brain. During the fMRI scans, the participants engaged in four different exercises: resting and letting their minds wander, recalling detailed memories, and entering two distinct hypnotic states.

Among the highly hypnotizable individuals, three significant differences in brain activity were observed compared to those with low hypnotizability. Firstly, there was reduced activity in a region called the dorsal anterior cingulate cortex, which is involved in self-awareness and information processing. This reduced activity suggests that during hypnosis, individuals become absorbed and less concerned with external distractions.

Secondly, there was increased connectivity between different parts of the salience network, including the dorsolateral prefrontal cortex and insula. The insula plays a role in various functions such as body control, emotions, empathy, and time perception, while the dorsolateral prefrontal cortex is involved in cognition, memory, and decision-making. Strengthening the connection between these regions may help the brain regulate and process information related to the body and its experiences during hypnosis.

Lastly, there was reduced connectivity between the dorsolateral prefrontal cortex and the default mode network, which is active when the mind is at rest or engaged in self-referential thinking. This decoupling allows individuals to perform actions without excessive self-consciousness, enabling behavioral changes suggested by the therapist to occur more smoothly.

Understanding how hypnosis affects the brain can have significant implications for developing more effective treatments, especially for individuals who are less responsive to hypnosis. Brain stimulation techniques could potentially be used in conjunction with hypnosis to enhance its therapeutic benefits. While the research is still in its early stages, identifying the specific brain areas and connections involved in hypnosis marks a significant step towards this goal.

The influence of hypnosis on the brain is evident, regardless of whether one believes in its efficacy. Neuroscientists have observed measurable changes in brain activity and connectivity during hypnotic states. For example, studies have shown that hypnotized individuals experience reduced pain sensitivity

Chapter 3: Enhancing Your Sleep Quality

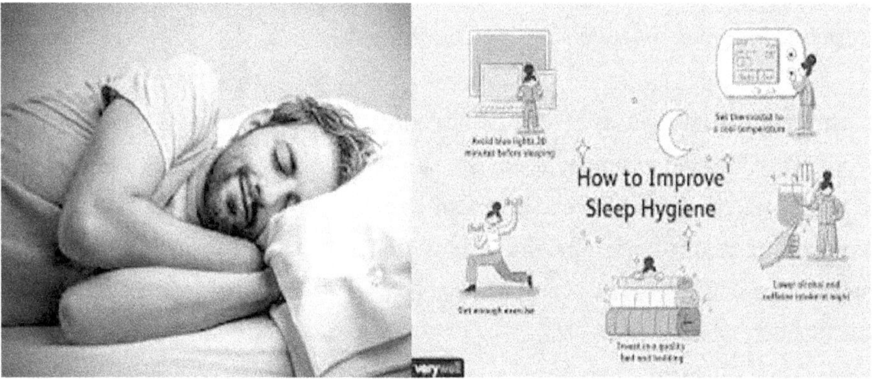

To achieve optimal daytime well-being, it is crucial to prioritize a good night's sleep. For individuals who struggle to obtain sufficient rest each night, there are numerous tips that can be tried to enhance the chances of falling asleep and improve the quality of sleep. Consider the following simple suggestions to promote better sleep:

Minimize Screen Time: In today's smartphone-dominated era, it is essential to address the detrimental impact of excessive screen usage on our sleep patterns. Although technology advancements have made our lives easier, they do not contribute positively to our sleep quality. Sleep should not be regarded as a passive state, but rather as a crucial period for our overall well-being, allowing our bodies to undergo necessary tissue repairs and growth. Excessive screen exposure poses serious consequences for our health.

To counter this, it is recommended to shut down your phone at night. This practice enables faster sleep onset, better quality of rest, and a more refreshed awakening by eliminating disruptive signals and vibrations throughout the night. Keep your phone at least 3 feet away from your body to minimize the effects of electromagnetic radiation. If you use your phone as an alarm, placing it farther away will safeguard your well-being and compel you to get up and turn it off in the morning. Limit unnecessary phone usage and avoid disconnecting from the world around you. Engage in genuine human interactions, cultivate close relationships, and appreciate your surroundings. By actively participating in your environment and looking up from your screens, you may discover fascinating things.

Dim Bright Lights in the Evening: Bright lights in the evening can deceive your body into perceiving it as daytime, reducing the production of melatonin, a hormone essential for relaxation and deep sleep. To create a more serene environment, opt for lamps, dimmer switches, or candles. Two hours before bedtime, turn off the TV, computer, and other electronic devices.

Prioritize Physical Fitness: Given the prevalence of sedentary lifestyles, especially due to work obligations, incorporating exercise into our routines is the initial step toward becoming smarter sleepers. When done correctly, exercise can facilitate quicker sleep onset and improved sleep quality. Physical activity aids in reducing cortisol levels, known as the "stress hormone," which responds to physical stress on the body.

Exercise also establishes a foundation for natural rest by promoting deep and lasting relaxation. It helps calm us down, rejuvenate the nervous system, enhance blood circulation, and reduce anxiety levels. Engaging in light workouts, stretching, household chores, or running in the evening can facilitate early sleep onset and improve sleep quality. However, it is advisable to avoid vigorous exercise close to bedtime, as it may hinder falling asleep properly.

Avoid Late-Day Caffeine Consumption: Consuming caffeine, a stimulant, should be avoided four to six hours before bedtime. Caffeine is present in coffee, iced tea, chocolate, and various over-the-counter medications. For instance, having two cups of coffee during dinner and some chocolate ice cream can result in a substantial caffeine intake of around 500 milligrams. It is also worth noting that caffeine can remain in your system for up to 12 hours. Opt for decaffeinated coffee after dinner.

Steer Clear of Cigarettes and Alcohol in the Evening: Similarly, it is advisable to abstain from nicotine intake close to bedtime, as nicotine acts as a stimulant and disrupts sleep. Smoking before bed, despite the initial feeling of relaxation, introduces stimulants into your bloodstream. Reduce nicotine intake before bed by smoking fewer cigarettes in the four hours leading up to bedtime, and abstain completely for at least 30 minutes before sleep.

Alcohol, though it may facilitate falling asleep initially, tends to cause disturbances and awakenings during the night

Chapter 4: Understanding REM and Non-REM Sleep

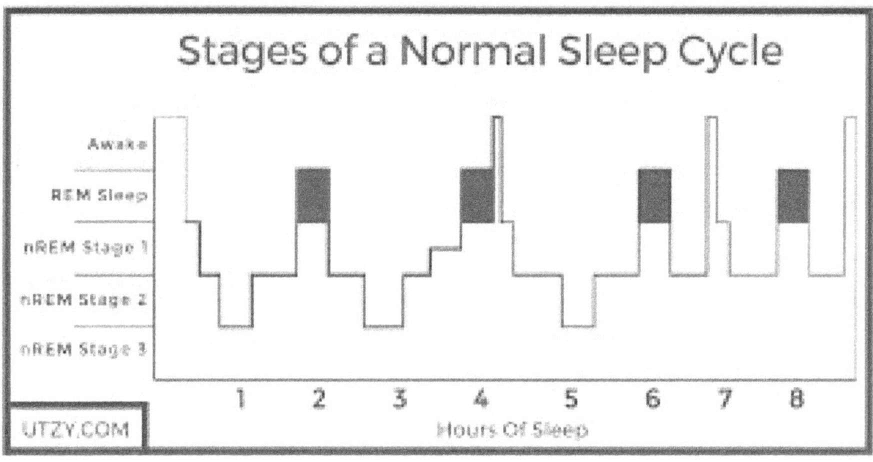

Phases Explained Throughout a typical night's sleep, we go through different stages of sleep, each with its own significance in the sleep process. These stages lead us to the deepest stage called REM (Rapid Eye Movement), where dreaming and subconscious functioning occur. While all four stages are equally important for restful sleep, it is during REM sleep that we experience the most profound subconscious activity.

Sleep Stage 1: Light Sleep Phase The initial stage is characterized as the lightest phase of sleep, during which we can easily be awakened or disturbed.

In this stage, we feel drowsy, exhibit slow eye movements, and may doze off briefly before awakening again. Our body relaxes, and we may experience muscle contractions or a falling sensation. Brain activity starts to slow down as we gradually drift into sleep, preparing for deeper rest.

Sleep Stage 2: Non-REM Sleep During the second stage, also known as the first phase of deep sleep, brain activity continues to decrease. Body temperature lowers, and heart rate slows down. Eye movements remain sluggish, occasionally interrupted by brief periods of rapid eye movement called sleep spindles. These spindles, along with bursts of brain activity known as "K complexes," are visible as spikes on brain activity charts during sleep studies. Although the exact purpose of these events is still being studied, they seem to play a role in protecting sleep continuity by alternating between slow eye movements and the other two events.

Sleep Stage 3: Deeper Non-REM Sleep The third stage, also referred to as deep or restorative sleep, deepens further compared to the previous stage. It becomes increasingly challenging to awaken someone during this phase due to the presence of slow (delta) waves. People tend to remain relatively stable in stage 3, transitioning into the deepest level of sleep. This stage is highly satisfying and contributes to feeling well-rested and functioning optimally. When we miss a night of sleep, the subsequent night's sleep compensates by prolonging the duration of deep sleep to restore the deficit. This adjustment allows the body to skip or reduce the earlier stages of sleep when more deep sleep is required.

Sleep Stage 4: REM (Rapid Eye Movement) REM sleep is characterized by rapid eye movement and high brain activity levels, comparable to wakefulness. It is the stage during which dreaming takes place. Sleepwalking, talking, or night terrors are more likely to occur in this deep stage of sleep. Upon waking up in the morning, we are typically in the REM stage. If we wake up abruptly during REM sleep, especially from a vivid dream, it may feel like an abrupt interruption. This stage is often associated with dream recall. Insufficient deep sleep can lead to mental fogginess and grogginess upon transitioning from sleep to wakefulness.

Importance of Waking Up During the Light Sleep Phase, Not Deep Sleep To fully benefit from a night's rest, it is crucial to progress through all four sleep stages, eventually reaching REM sleep after deep sleep. Although many individuals wake up during the REM stage, it may not result in the most refreshing experience. They may feel groggy and struggle to wake up immediately. Some people try to compensate by increasing their sleep duration, believing that more time spent asleep will prevent waking up in this state. However, waking up during the REM stage can still occur even after eight or more hours of sleep. To ensure a more refreshing and satisfying awakening, it is recommended to wake up during the light sleep phase, such as the first stage. This simple solution promotes a good night's rest. However, determining the ideal waking time can be challenging due to busy schedules and limited sleep hours.

Chapter 5: Understanding the Mechanisms of Hypnosis in the Brain

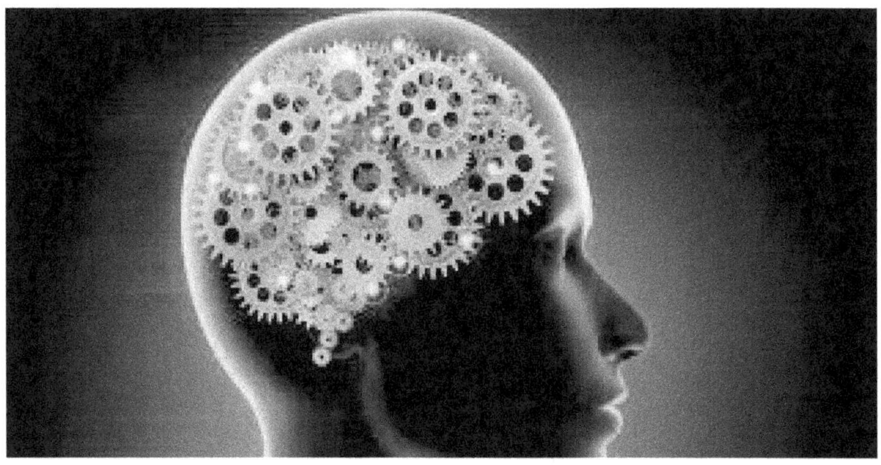

Regardless of one's belief in the effectiveness of hypnosis, neuroscientists are now presenting evidence that this practice does have measurable effects on the brain. In a study conducted in Germany, it was discovered that individuals under hypnosis experienced a significant reduction in pain sensitivity when exposed to painful stimuli. Using functional magnetic resonance imaging (fMRI), researchers also observed distinct patterns of brain activity in hypnotized subjects compared to non-hypnotized subjects who received the same painful stimuli.

One interesting finding from the study was that areas associated with color processing in the brain remained active even when hypnotized subjects were presented with black and white photographs instead of color images. Most of these studies have noted that the effects of hypnosis on the brain are most pronounced in individuals considered highly suggestible. Skeptics argue that these highly suggestible volunteers are predisposed to believe in things like hypnosis and, therefore, experience a self-induced placebo effect when they believe they are hypnotized.

However, a recent study conducted by researchers at the University of Virginia revealed that individuals who were highly susceptible to hypnosis exhibited significant differences in their brain structures. On average, these individuals had a larger platform, a part of the brain associated with attention and the transfer of information between prefrontal cortices.

Scientific research demonstrates that hypnosis, despite its skeptics, is capable of producing measurable changes in the human brain. As one enters a hypnotic state, characterized by slow breathing, relaxed muscles, and a weightless feeling, brain activity also undergoes specific alterations. Researchers in the United States studied the brains of 57 individuals during guided hypnosis and observed specific changes in activity and connectivity within certain brain regions involved in mind-body interactions.

The findings, published in the journal Cerebral Cortex, may provide valuable insights for clinicians to better utilize hypnosis as a therapeutic tool, particularly for pain control. Hypnosis has shown promise in treating various conditions such as phobias, post-traumatic stress disorder (PTSD), obesity, and depression during childbirth.

A typical hypnosis session begins with a discussion between the patient and the therapist about the goals of the session. The patient is then guided into a relaxed state of focus, during which the therapist reinforces the goals through verbal suggestions, and the patient may visualize and imagine them.

In highly hypnotizable individuals, such sessions have proven effective in reducing chronic pain and aiding in smoking cessation. However, the exact processes occurring in the brain during hypnosis remain unclear.

To shed light on this, researchers at Stanford University conducted a study to investigate brain activity during hypnosis. They screened 545 healthy individuals for hypnotizability and selected 36 highly hypnotizable subjects and 21 individuals with low hypnotizability scores. The subjects' brain activity was measured using functional magnetic resonance imaging (fMRI) while they engaged in various mental activities, including resting, recalling memories, and entering hypnotic states.

Comparing the highly hypnotizable group with the less susceptible group, researchers identified three significant differences in brain activity. Firstly, the highly hypnotizable individuals exhibited reduced activity in the dorsal anterior cingulate cortex, a brain region involved in attention regulation and information processing. This decreased activity indicated a higher level of absorption and reduced awareness of external stimuli during hypnosis.

Secondly, the connectivity between the dorsolateral prefrontal cortex and insula, which are involved in body control, emotion, and time perception, was enhanced in the highly hypnotizable group. This increased connectivity may facilitate the brain's ability to regulate and process bodily sensations during hypnosis.

Lastly, there was reduced connectivity between the dorsolateral prefrontal cortex and the default mode network in highly hypnotizable individuals. The default mode network is active when the mind is wandering, self-reflect

Chapter 6: Sleep Learning System

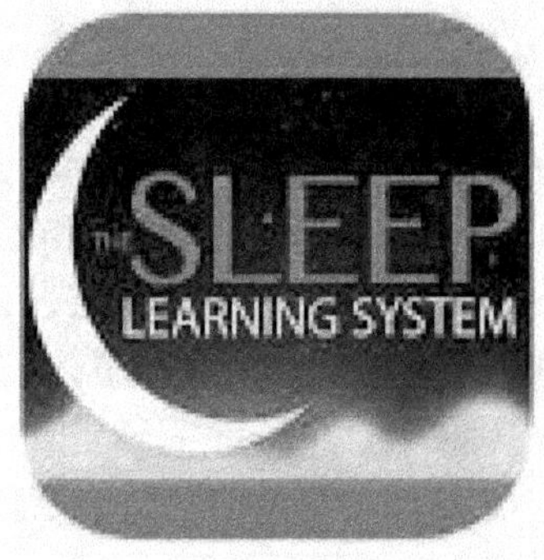

Understanding the Sleep Learning System

Summary: Transforming night into day is not particularly beneficial. While each person's sleep needs are unique, there are distinguishable phases of deep and shallow sleep. The architecture of sleep reveals that the first half of the night is predominantly deep sleep, while the second half consists of more light, shallow sleep or slumber.

Paraphrase of "Dive-In Dream":

The process of falling asleep can be compared to focusing our internal energy or attention. We've all experienced the tiredness that comes from reading, where our consciousness narrows and our gaze freezes before we drift into deeper realms and eventually fall asleep. Falling asleep is essentially entering a trance-like state, which is an innate ability we possess, even before birth. Various techniques and strategies outlined in Parts I and II of this guide can help us achieve this trance state quickly. By following these processes, we can fully relax and minimize external factors that may disrupt our sleep patterns.

Paraphrase of "What Happens When We Finally Go To Sleep? Where Does Our Consciousness Go?":

In the realm of consciousness, valuable insights have been gained from the study of Eastern traditions like Hinduism and Buddhism, which have delved into these matters for centuries or even millennia. These traditions propose the existence of a comprehensive consciousness referred to as "Buddha consciousness." By awakening to this level of consciousness and maintaining self-awareness, one can recognize the interconnectedness and inseparability of everything in the world. The phase of deep sleep seems to bring us closest to this state, where maintaining clarity of consciousness can lead to genuine bliss. Buddhist Zen masters and others suggest that within the deepest peace of this state, profound energy for development and healing resides, offering a significantly enhanced perspective on the significance of deep sleep.

Paraphrase of "The Phases Of Rest And Activity":

Using electroencephalograph recordings of brain waves, researchers have shed light on the phenomenon of relaxation states. The first half of the night is primarily dedicated to body regeneration through deep sleep, while the second half focuses on the sensory and spiritual integration of the body through BDG-dream. Researchers have identified four distinct phases of consciousness and regeneration induced by the human brain. The transition from waking consciousness (characterized by relatively chaotic beta waves) to sleep involves a progression from calmer alpha waves to slower theta waves, ultimately leading to delta waves, indicating deep sleep. This sequence repeats in reverse order approximately every hour and a half, with the occurrence of the BDG phase, which exhibits wave characteristics similar to wakefulness. Typically, we go through four to five sleep phases every hour and a half, forming a fundamental pattern of our night's rest. Each individual's "sleep profile" exhibits unique characteristics.

Paraphrase of "Sleep Regulators":

Sleep is regulated by an internal clock situated in the brain, dictating the rhythm of sleep and wakefulness. This rhythm remains largely unaffected, even in the face of sleep disturbances.

Paraphrase of "How Long Should You Sleep?":

The duration of sleep a person requires is a subject of various theories backed by increasing scientific evidence. Just as people can be classified based on their dietary preferences, their need for sleep can also vary. Most individuals feel their best after seven to eight hours of sleep, but many fail to obtain this necessary amount. Alarm clocks often interrupt their natural waking process, leaving them feeling unwell if they manage to sleep for less than six hours. Studies suggest that surpassing ten hours of sleep is unnecessary for adults. Children, however, may require ten to eleven hours of sleep, and their sleep needs can also differ according to type. For many people, an ideal combination might involve a relatively short night's rest supplemented with several brief sleep

Chapter 7: Achieving Faster Sleep and Improving Sleep Quality

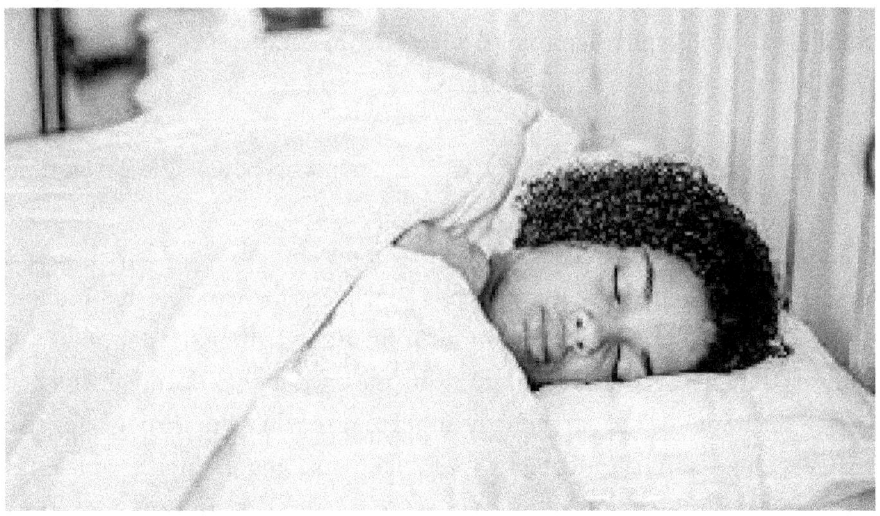

Getting adequate and high-quality sleep has a profound impact on a person's mood, attitude, and overall performance. Improved sleep contributes to better physical well-being, bolstering the immune system, lung function, heart health, and skin condition. Essentially, when you sleep well, everything in life tends to be better.

Conversely, a disrupted sleep pattern is detrimental, leading to irritability, diminished performance, and various health problems. It increases susceptibility to stress and other health-related issues.

Fortunately, there are numerous strategies to ensure a restful night's sleep. Creating an optimal sleep environment is key, characterized by a comfortable bed, pillows, fresh bedding, a quiet and dimly lit space, free of clutter, and kept cool. Meeting these standards is crucial for a good sleep environment.

Sometimes, sleep troubles stem from poor habits rather than the environment alone. Establishing consistent sleep and wake times is essential. It is also crucial to minimize mental stimulation at least an hour before bedtime, develop a bedtime routine to unwind gradually, avoid alcoholic beverages within three hours of sleeping, and have meals two to three hours before sleep. Additionally, removing electronic devices such as computers and phones from the bedroom promotes peaceful sleep.

But what if these methods do not work? Can hypnosis be a potential solution?

Understanding how hypnosis aids sleep is important. You may have heard of the counting sheep technique, which is a form of self-hypnosis that induces sleep. When falling asleep, the mind transitions from external reality to internal thoughts, generating images from the imaginative and dream-related part of the brain. By encouraging the mind to make this shift through positive imagery, sleep can be induced. It is crucial to use imagination for pleasant thoughts rather than worrying, as worrying triggers the production of stress hormones, making the body more alert and defeating the purpose of sleep induction.

Hypnosis is a valuable tool for promoting relaxation and quieting the conscious mind, making it beneficial for individuals struggling with sleep issues. It is not limited to counting sheep but encompasses various techniques. For instance, a guided relaxation journey can be used, where one envisions walking on a beautiful beach, feeling the light breeze and sand on the feet. Alternatively, a serene stroll in a splendid garden with colorful blooming flowers, birds singing, and leaves rustling in the wind can be imagined. The key is to immerse oneself in a pleasant mental setting, experiencing the sensations vividly. As relaxation sets in, one can transition to the internal reality, initiating a peaceful and rejuvenating sleep.

Another technique involves visualizing colors. Starting with the color red and progressing through the spectrum to violet, one can imagine objects or elements associated with each color. By reaching violet, a state of readiness for a deep and healthy sleep is achieved. This technique can be employed during hypnosis sessions, where the individual visualizes the colors and reinforces the intention to sleep.

In conclusion, falling asleep quickly and improving sleep quality are crucial for overall well-being. Creating an optimal sleep environment, adopting healthy sleep habits, and incorporating hypnosis techniques can all contribute to achieving a peaceful and rejuvenating sleep experience.

Chapter 8: Enhancing Deep Sleep

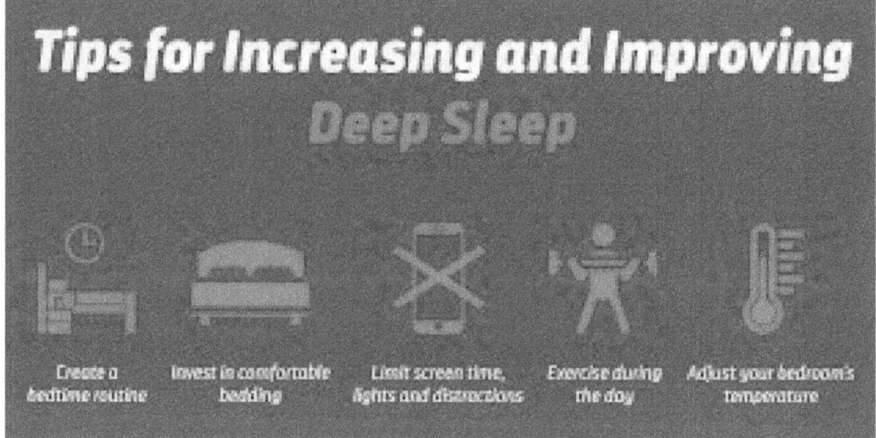

Sleep plays a crucial role in our lives, and it involves more than meets the eye. If you struggle with falling asleep, getting enough sleep, or dealing with an injury, there are factors beyond simply lying down that can affect your sleep. The position in which you sleep can significantly impact the quality of your sleep, indicating that finding the right sleep posture might be beneficial.

Different sleep positions offer various advantages. Changing your sleep position can be helpful if you have health issues or experience pain. While it may not be an overnight fix, gradually training your body to sleep in a new position can be essential for improving sleep quality. However, don't stress if you're uncomfortable with changing your position entirely. Modifying your existing sleep position can also yield benefits.

Types of Sleep Positions

Everyone has unique needs, so understanding what works best for your body and sleep is crucial. Here are some of the recommended sleeping positions:

Flat on your back: Although not the most popular position (only 8% of people sleep on their backs), sleeping on your back offers significant health benefits. It allows your spine, neck, and head to rest in a neutral position, promoting proper alignment. This position can alleviate pain by reducing pressure on your back and joints. Additionally, it helps prevent acid reflux when you elevate your head using a pillow. However, sleeping on your back may obstruct breathing and worsen snoring, especially for individuals with sleep apnea. Placing a pillow under your knees or propping yourself up with an extra pillow can relieve pressure on the spine and aid breathing.

Fetal position: The fetal position is the most popular sleeping position, with approximately forty-one percent of people favoring it. This position involves sleeping on your side, preferably the left side, with your knees bent and torso slightly curled. It is particularly beneficial for pregnant individuals as it prevents pressure on the liver and improves blood circulation. However, sleeping tightly in the fetal position may hinder deep breathing and cause morning soreness, especially for those with joint issues. Loosening the position by straightening your body and placing a pillow between your knees can make it more comfortable.

Side sleeping: Sleeping on your side, with your torso and legs relatively straight, can be advantageous. This position helps maintain spinal elongation, preventing back and neck pain. It also aids in reducing heartburn, acid reflux, and snoring while promoting better digestion. Studies suggest switching sides at night to prevent acid reflux and heartburn. However, side sleeping may cause jaw tightness, shoulder stiffness, and facial wrinkles. Placing a pillow between your legs can align your hips and prevent lower back pain.

Stomach sleeping: Sleeping on your stomach is the least common position, with only 7% of adults preferring it. While it can be beneficial for sleep apnea and snoring, this position offers no additional advantages. It is challenging to maintain a neutral spine position, potentially leading to back and neck pain. Furthermore, stomach sleeping exerts unnecessary pressure on joints and muscles, resulting in discomfort and nerve irritation. If stomach sleeping is necessary, keeping your face down instead of turning it to one side can help keep your airways open. Using a thin pillow under your head can alleviate neck stress, and placing a pillow beneath your lower belly or pelvis can reduce lower back pain.

Free-fall position: Approximately seventeen percent of the population chooses the free-fall position, lying on their stomachs with their arms beneath or around the pillow and their heads turned to one side.

Choosing Your Sleep Position

Consider the following factors before settling into your preferred sleep position:

Appearance: Sleeping on your stomach or side can cause facial creases over time, potentially leading to chronic skin changes or breakouts

Chapter 9: Serene Imagery Visualizing a Peaceful Ocean Retreat

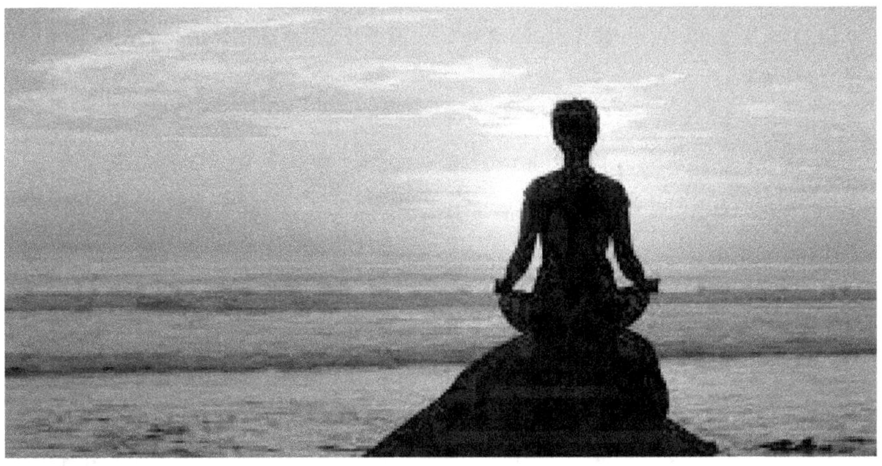

Prepare for a tranquil evening ahead. Before you surrender to sleep, let me transport you to the most exquisite beach you can imagine. This serene place will envelop you in relaxation and soothe your very essence.

Start by taking a deep breath and settling into a comfortable position. Rest your head on the soft pillow and take another deep breath, allowing your body to relax and your muscles to loosen.

Good…

Continue to release any lingering tension from your body with each breath. Inhale slowly, then exhale with a gentle whooshing sound, mimicking the rhythmic crash of waves on the sandy shore.

With every breath, feel yourself becoming increasingly relaxed. Breathe in deeply, pause for a moment, and then let go. Sense your body releasing all tension, completely surrendering to the calm and peaceful rhythm of your breath.

Imagine a gentle wave of relaxation coursing through your entire being, just like the ebb and flow of the ocean's majestic waves. It starts at your toes and flows upward, traveling through your legs, torso, arms, and even your head. With each passing breath, every part of your body succumbs to deep relaxation.

Inhale slowly and deeply once more, releasing the air with a gentle whoosh, while conjuring the image of a pristine white sand beach in your mind.

Picture yourself standing on this beach, feeling the warm and velvety sand beneath your feet. The turquoise waves of the ocean in front of you create a soothing whooshing sound, akin to your breath. Surrounding this beach is a tropical forest, alive with the melodious songs of beautiful birds. The palm tree leaves rustle gently in the wind, and you can hear the symphony of crickets and tropical frogs harmonizing in the rainforest.

Take notice of the vibrant greens of nature, marveling at how each leaf reflects the sunlight with its unique beauty. Feel the gentle warmth of the sun caressing your skin, embracing you in its calming embrace. This place embodies tranquility.

As you gaze at the ocean, you'll notice that the water is shallow near the shore, gradually transitioning into a rich sapphire blue on the distant horizon. Above, fluffy white clouds drift lazily across the sky, resembling the raw blossom of cotton. The sun's rays intermittently warm your skin as they peek through the passing clouds.

In the vicinity, you spot a spacious opening in the rocks, beckoning you to explore. As you step inside the cave, the sound of ocean waves bouncing off the rocky walls amplifies, creating a magnificent symphony. The cave itself is a sight to behold. Trickling water leads you to its source, where fresh water springs from the rocks, producing the most soothing sound of moving water you've ever heard. Even without sunlight, the water in the cave shimmers with an ethereal glow.

Scoop some of this pure and refreshing water into your cupped hands and take a sip. Its taste is unparalleled, nourishing and revitalizing every part of your being. Tropical birds, aware of this hidden water source, fly into the cave, chirping their melodious songs. They drink from the various puddles that have formed on the cave floor, dipping their beaks into the water and letting it trickle down their throats. Curiously, they regard you as if you're part of their flock.

These magnificent birds come so close that you can admire the stunning rainbow of colors adorning their feathers—bright reds, yellows, greens, and turquoise blues that match the ocean's waters. The crisp white surrounding their eyes adds to their beauty, and they gaze at you with kindness and curiosity.

Chapter 10: Conscious Consumption

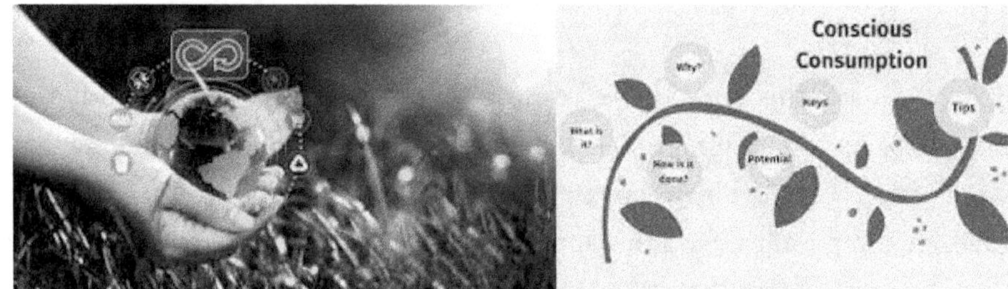

The Significance of Sleep and a Clear Conscience

Summary: In this chapter, the importance of sleep and a clear conscience is emphasized. Despite the lack of scientific understanding of why sleep is necessary, it is universally recognized that adequate rest is vital for a healthy life. Sleep deprivation can lead to various issues, including hallucinations and impaired daily functioning. Research suggests that good sleep contributes to overall health and longevity, with women often outliving men due to their better sleep quality. However, in today's modern society, many individuals prioritize material wealth and power over quality sleep, which can hinder their ability to attain sound rest. This chapter explores the connection between sleep, consciousness, and the four stages of reality described in Indian scriptures. It highlights the significance of deep sleep, the soul's equilibrium, and the benefits of a restful night's sleep in rejuvenating the body and mind. While sleep remains a mystery to scientists, its numerous benefits are acknowledged, such as energy restoration, tissue repair, and the opportunity for the mind and soul to address unresolved issues. Furthermore, it emphasizes that a troubled conscience cannot find solace in sleep, leading to insomnia and lasting damage. Ultimately, the chapter emphasizes the incomparable value of sound sleep and a clear conscience in maintaining a healthy and fulfilling life, surpassing any material gains obtained through disregarding one's moral compass.

Chapter 11: Achieving Instant Sleep through Meditation and the Power of Napping

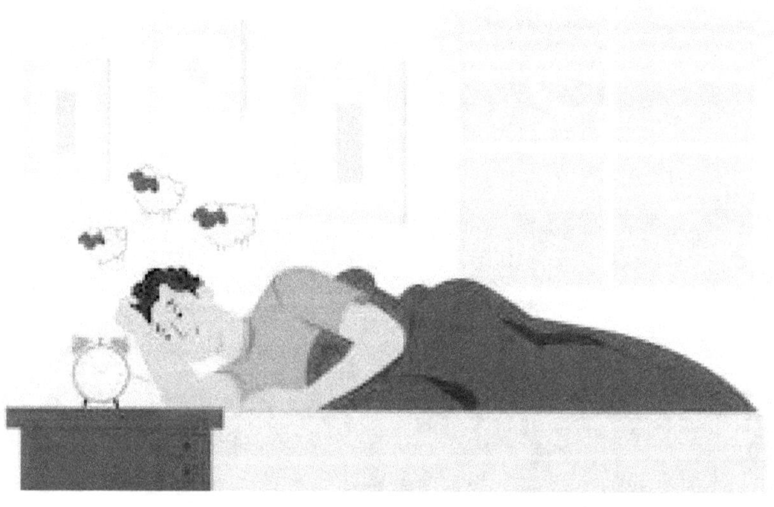

Synopsis: This chapter explores the concept of using meditation techniques and power naps to fall asleep quickly and reap various benefits. A power nap is a short sleep that ends before entering deep sleep, and although it may not provide the same restfulness as a full night's sleep, it can enhance creativity, problem-solving abilities, and memory. The guide suggests finding the most suitable time for a power nap that aligns with one's schedule and avoiding napping when alertness is necessary. Naps exceeding 30 minutes can lead to deep sleep, so setting an alarm is crucial. Even short naps as brief as five minutes can enhance daytime well-being and memory. Early napping during the first 12 hours of the day can aid nighttime sleep. Conversely, napping late in the day may disrupt nighttime rest. The chapter also addresses the optimal duration of naps, emphasizing that they are intended to provide refreshment rather than deep sleep. Naps can range from as little as 5 minutes to a maximum of 90 minutes, especially for those who are sleep-deprived. The importance of setting an alarm to prevent oversleeping is emphasized. The chapter includes scripts for different nap durations, focusing on relaxation techniques and visualization to induce a state of restfulness. The scripts guide individuals to relax their bodies, calm their minds, and imagine tranquil environments to facilitate sleep. The chapter concludes by highlighting the benefits of power naps and quick rest meditation in rejuvenating the mind and body, leading to increased productivity and a refreshed state upon waking up.

Chapter 12: Tips for Better Sleep

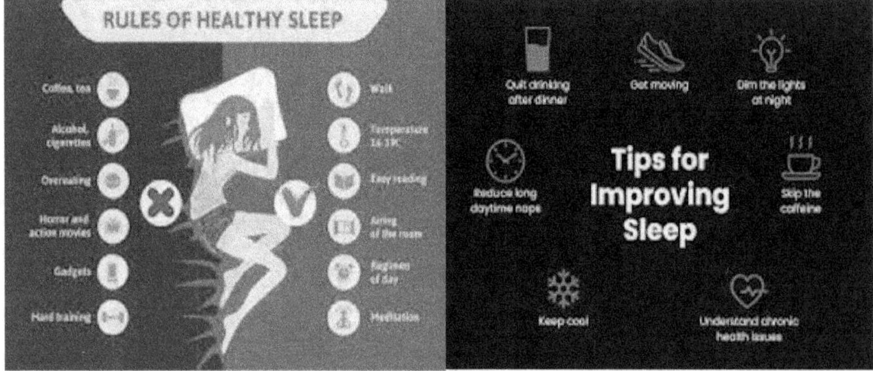

To ensure a good night's sleep and overall well-being, it's important to follow some simple rules before bedtime. Here are some easy tips to consider:

Reduce screen time: In today's technological age, excessive screen exposure can negatively impact sleep quality. Minimize the use of electronic devices, especially before bed, to improve your sleep. Keep your phone away from your body, check it only when necessary, and engage in real-life experiences.

Turn off bright lights in the evening: Bright lights can disrupt your body's natural sleep patterns. Opt for dimmer lighting or use lamps and candles to create a more serene environment. Avoid using electronic devices like TVs and computers at least two hours before bedtime.

Maintain physical fitness: Regular exercise can help you fall asleep faster and improve sleep quality. Engage in light physical activities or stretching in the evening to calm your body and reduce anxiety. Avoid intense workouts close to bedtime.

Avoid consuming caffeine late in the day: Stimulants like caffeine can interfere with sleep. Refrain from consuming caffeine-containing beverages or foods, such as coffee, tea, chocolate, or certain medications, at least four to six hours before bedtime.

Avoid cigarettes and alcohol in the evening: Nicotine is a stimulant that can disrupt sleep, while alcohol may cause waking up during the night. Minimize or avoid smoking and drinking alcohol close to bedtime for better sleep quality.

Don't eat heavy meals in the evening: Large or spicy meals can cause discomfort and hormone disruption, affecting your sleep. Opt for light snacks if you're hungry a few hours before bed.

Optimize your bedroom environment: Create a sleep-friendly environment by reducing distractions. Keep your bedroom cool, quiet, and dark. Use eye shades, blackout curtains, earplugs, and other devices to enhance your sleep environment.

Keep pets out of bed and bedroom: While pets are great companions, their presence in bed can disrupt your sleep. Provide a comfortable space for your pets outside of the bedroom and establish a sleep schedule that doesn't involve them.

Sleep on a comfortable mattress and pillows: Ensure your bed and pillows provide adequate comfort and support. Choose a mattress and pillows that suit your preferred sleeping position to maintain proper spinal alignment.

Maintain cleanliness: Keep your sleep environment clean and free from allergens like dust. Dust and clean your room regularly to minimize allergies and create a healthier sleep environment.

Shower before sleep: Taking a warm bath or shower before bedtime can promote relaxation and improve sleep quality. Aim for a shower or bath approximately 1-2 hours before sleep, keeping the duration under 10 minutes.

Clear your mind and relax in the evening: Engage in relaxation techniques such as listening to calming music, reading, meditating, or deep breathing to quiet your mind and reduce stress before bed.

Make a list for tomorrow: Jot down your tasks for the next day to declutter your mind and relieve the burden of remembering everything before sleep. Spend a few minutes before bed to create a to-do list for better mental relaxation.

Do remaining tasks later: Avoid engaging in work-related activities or stressful discussions before bed. Turn off the TV and log out of social media accounts to allow your mind to unwind.

Don't make efforts to sleep: If you find your mind racing and unable to sleep, don't force it. Engage in relaxing activities until you feel tired. Avoid trying too hard to sleep, as it can be counterproductive.

By implementing these healthy sleep habits and finding what works best for you, you can improve the quality of your sleep and overall well-being.

Chapter 13: Stop Overthinking, Anxiety, and Stress with Hypnosis Script

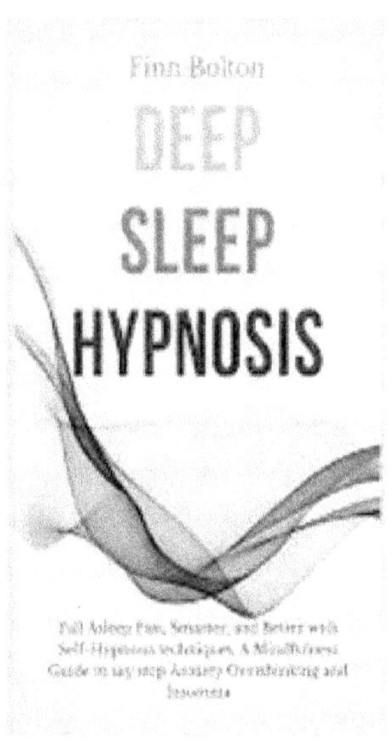

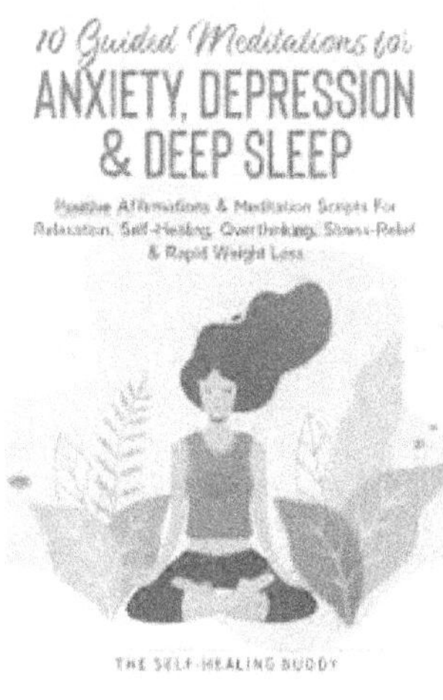

Currently, I would like to take you on an incredible journey and removing

Your tendency to analyze things too much. Firstly, let me draw your attention to my voice. Pay close attention to the powerful force

I speak to draw you to my voice. With each syllable I utter, this force becomes stronger.

Find a place to sit or lie down that is quiet and comfortable; either is fine. Open the windows to let in some fresh air while making sure no one disturbs you. Pay attention to the sounds around you and then return your attention to my speech. The only sounds you can hear right now are the sound of some soothing music and my voice.

Chapter 14: Daily Affirmations for Managing Stress, Anxiety, Mindfulness, Relaxation, Sleep Improvement, Success, and Happiness

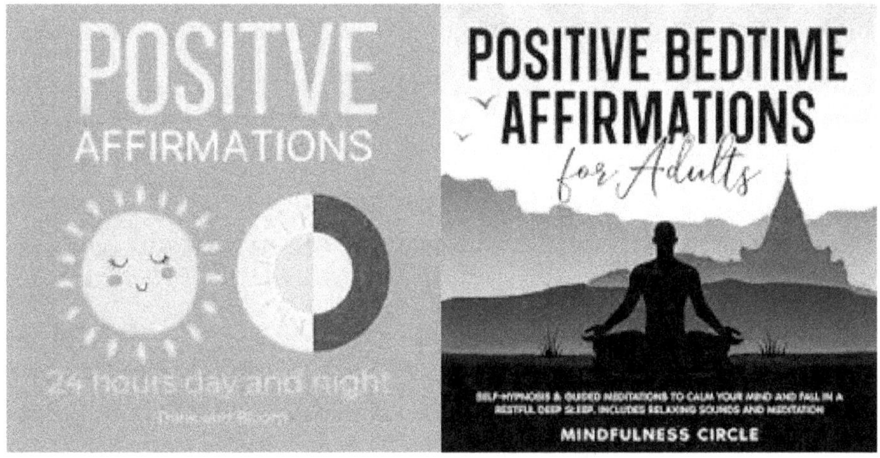

An affirmation is a statement you make to yourself to reinforce the importance of an idea. Throughout the day, you may find yourself thinking negative affirmations that validate your perspective, such as "I'm not good enough" or "Nothing is going right in my life." While these statements may not represent the whole truth, they can solidify a particular viewpoint.

To counteract negative affirmations and cultivate a more positive mindset, it's beneficial to focus on daily affirmations that are essential and helpful for achieving a restful night's sleep. Repeat these affirmations to yourself, write them down and place reminders around your home, or simply keep them in mind when you need them the most.

Incorporating physical activity can enhance the impact of affirmations. By combining a mental thought with a physical exercise, the affirmations become more tangible and easier to believe. One way to reinforce these affirmations is to hold a physical item while saying them, such as a small stone or a special pillow or blanket.

Breathing exercises can also be integrated with positive sleep affirmations. In addition to the common method of breathing in through the nose and out through the mouth, you can try breathing through alternate nostrils. By pairing these breathing techniques with affirmations, you can establish positive thinking patterns associated with the affirmations.

Keeping a journal dedicated to affirmations can be beneficial. Write down the affirmations that resonate with your life and experiences. Journaling about them helps you remember and identify the most effective ones for your well-being.

When you're having a challenging day, turn to these affirmations for a confidence boost and motivation. They are designed to support you in various aspects of life, including sleep, relaxation, and overall success.

Now let's begin reading the affirmations. Remember to focus on your breathing as we guide you through them. If you don't intend to fall asleep immediately, taking notes can also help.

Affirmations for Healthy Sleep:

I am committed to making healthy choices for my sleep habits. My daily actions affect my sleep quality, so I prioritize making the best choices for my overall well-being.

I embrace activities that contribute to my health, even if they are challenging. Restful sleep makes everything else in my life easier, and I recognize its importance.

Developing healthy habits is within my reach, and I dedicate my time to a better future.

Taking care of myself feels rewarding, and I deserve a good night's sleep along with all its benefits.

It's natural for me to require rest, and I choose to engage in healthy behaviors to improve my sleep cycles.

Dreams are a normal part of life, and I focus on embracing positive dreams while avoiding nightmares.

Going to bed at a suitable time benefits my health. Tomorrow's responsibilities will still be there, so ensuring adequate rest is crucial.

I value my body and strive to make choices that promote my individual well-being and lifestyle.

Nourishing my body with the right nutrients keeps me energized throughout the day.

Getting the right amount of sleep makes me strong, physically and mentally.

Quality sleep positively impacts my mental health, enhancing my overall well-being.

I am happier and more lighthearted when I've had a good night's sleep.

I am grateful for the opportunity to improve my sleep and overall health.

I appreciate my ability to make choices that benefit my health and well-being.

Habits are not inherently bad; I ensure that my habits promote a healthy lifestyle.

A good night's sleep reduces my stress levels. I am at my best when

Chapter 15: Techniques Of Guided Meditations For Sleep Anxiety

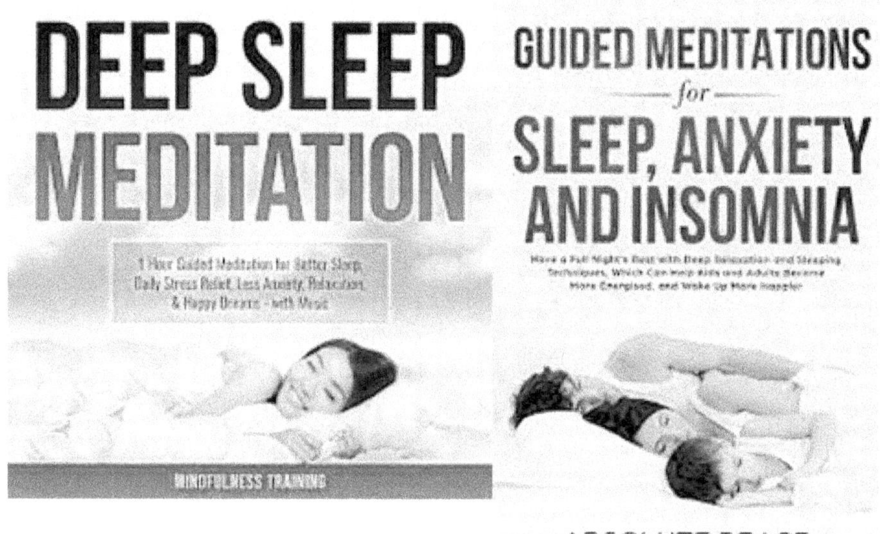

When you feel stiff or restless, you are likely experiencing anxiety.

Your heart may pulse more quickly and your

breathing might get faster. When they are concerned, some people can easily feel weak and exhausted.

It's crucial to recognize and recognize the contributions that your ideas contribute to your degree of worry. Anxiety is a result of thoughts, which are the images, memories, beliefs, judgments, and reflections that run through your mind. You can ask yourself: "What are the ideas and pictures in my head that maintain my current level of anxiety?"

It is also important to note that fear and anxiety will never solve your problems; instead, they will continue to worsen them. You may unknowingly be substituting practical actions.

Chapter 16: Learning To Drop Thoughts Effortlessly

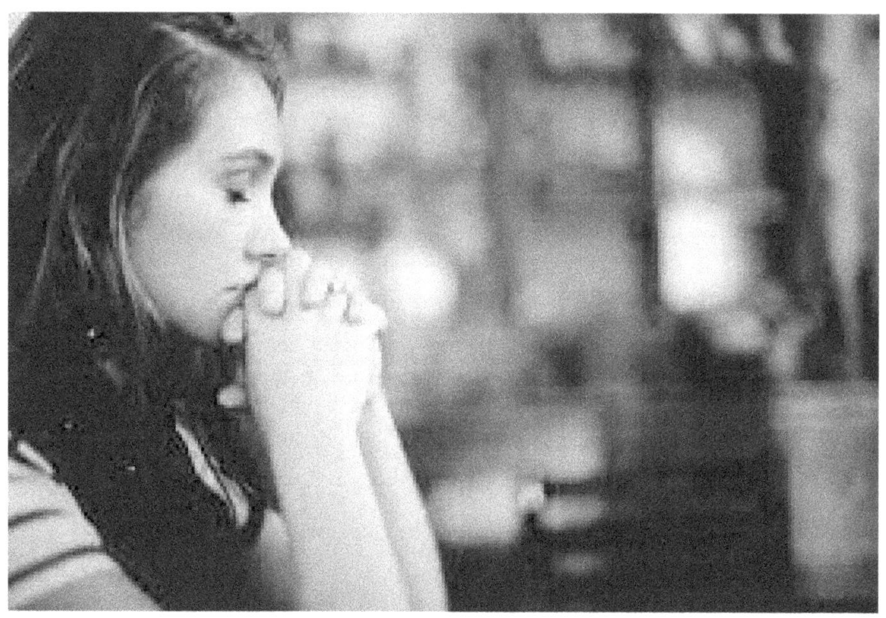

A Guided Meditation for Concentration

You need to set aside some time for meditation before you start this activity. Schedule some time for meditation. This

In this manner, none of your regular activities will conflict. In addition, be sure that the meditation period you set apart does not start just before an activity. Between your meditation and the next task, there should be at least a 15-minute rest.

Better still, pick the time of day when you can sleep the best. It can happen at sunset or when your shift comes to an end.

Keep in mind that we do not use the time here. What is best for you is our main priority.

Once you've determined the time that works best for you.

Chapter 17: Highly Successful Habits

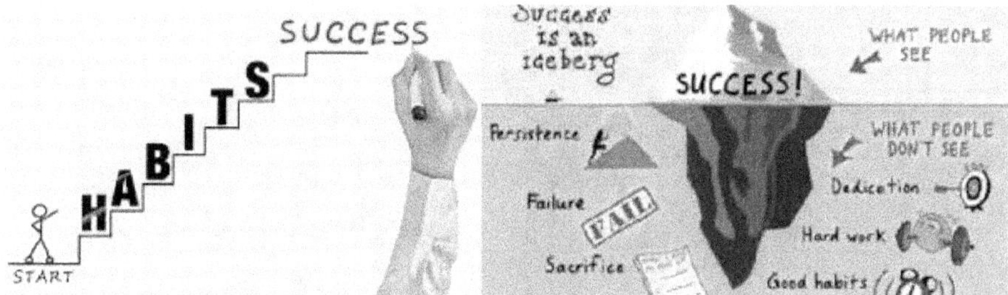

Regardless of how well you sleep, one main issue

Your way of life has changed, and there are many distractions in the bedroom. What do you need to do to go into this deep slumber

To make your room a peaceful space for meditation, you should get rid of all of them. This will be covered in more detail in the section that follows.

When you were a youngster, your parents may have put you on a nightly schedule to ensure that you got regular, deep sleep. Simply allowing you to utilize your bedroom for sleeping or taking a nap alone is a crucial component of this plan. Therefore, it requires that you remember that type of drill now that you are an adult.

Chapter 18: The First Steps to Ending the Insomnia Struggle

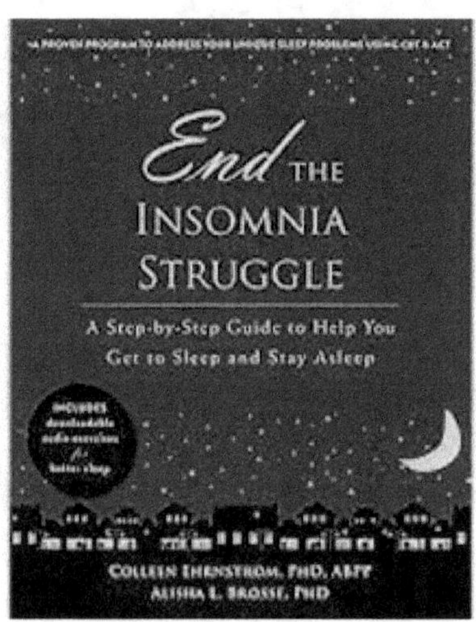

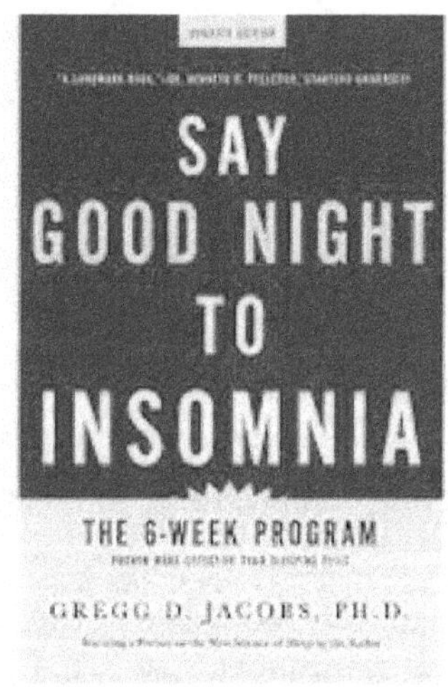

According to medical definitions, one of the major ailments is sleeplessness.

worldwide. Each day, more people report having insomnia. Around 29% of men, 37% of women, 25% of children, and 75% of youth in the world now are

This disease impacts expectant mothers. Sleep disruption is a symptom of insomnia. Patients don't always take their treatment for insomnia seriously and can just let things "go" on their own. As a result of this mentality, the disease develops into a chronic form, and neurological problems, internal organ pathologies, and mental disorders occur, all of which are uncomfortable and hazardous. Not everyone can manage their insomnia on their own, and in the majority of situations, professional medical assistance is required to attain a decent outcome.

Short version: Insomnia is a common occurrence.

Chapter 19: Deep Hypnosis Techniques

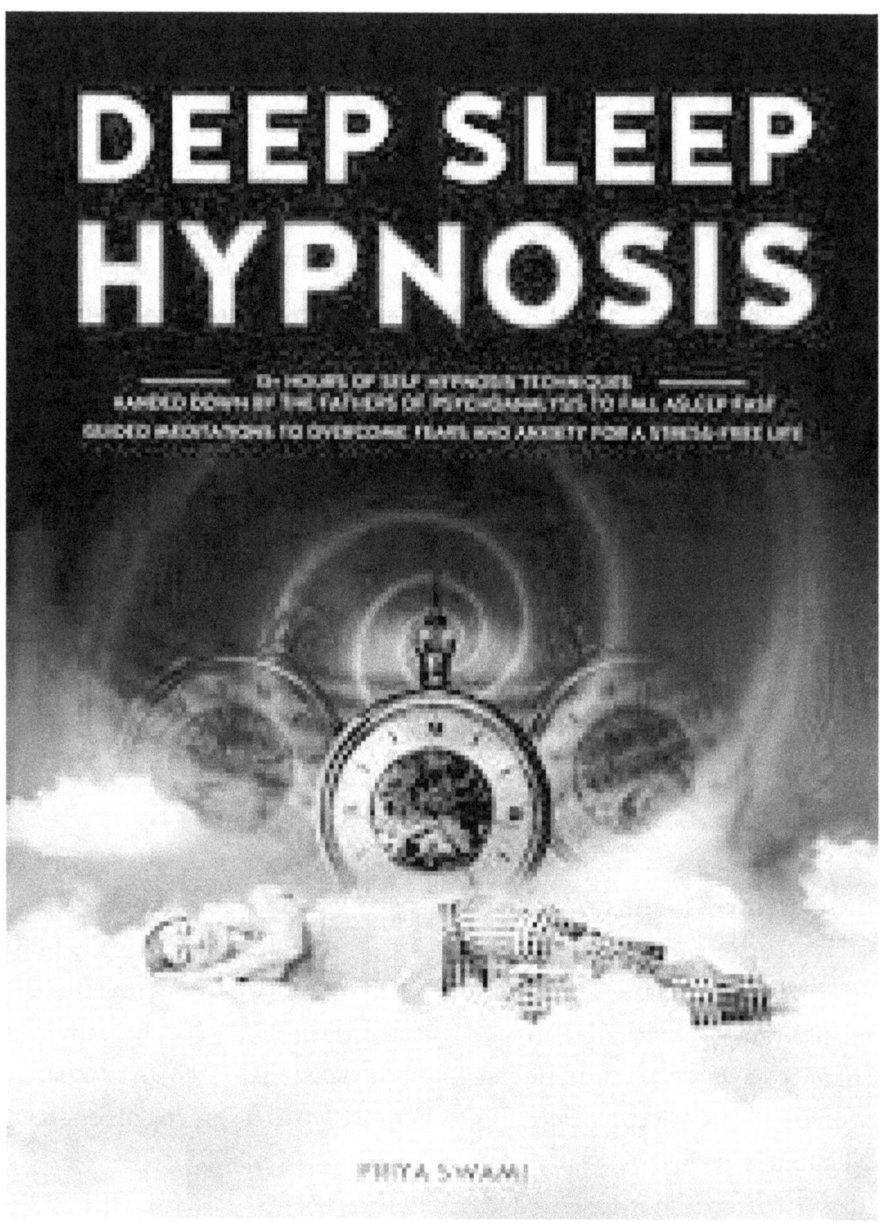

Insufficient sleep is a common problem in today's society, known as insomnia. Insomnia is characterized by the quality of sleep and the post-sleep feelings, rather than the duration or ease of falling asleep. Even if someone sleeps for eight hours a night but still feels fatigued and drowsy during the day, they may be experiencing insomnia, which can have various negative effects on health.

The causes of sleep deprivation and insomnia vary from person to person. Emotional factors such as anxiety, depression, and stress can contribute to insomnia. Other causes include traumatic experiences, medications affecting sleep, health issues interfering with sleep, excessive caffeine consumption, and an unfavorable sleep environment, among others. Understanding the causes and consequences of sleep deprivation is crucial in adopting practices that promote better sleep quality.

Meditation is a highly effective method for achieving deep sleep, and in this chapter, we will explore different meditation techniques for attaining restful sleep. Many individuals struggle to fall asleep at night, leading to daytime sleepiness, decreased productivity, and potential harm to overall health. However, research has shown that mindfulness meditation can help overcome this issue. Mindfulness meditation involves a mind-calming exercise focused on breathing and being fully present in the moment.

During mindfulness meditation, one concentrates on their breath and brings their attention to the present moment, avoiding thoughts about the past, present, or future. This practice helps break away from everyday thoughts and induces the relaxation response. It's important to note that mindfulness meditation is not meant to make you fall asleep immediately; rather, it enhances awareness and understanding of your mind, which ultimately promotes better sleep. Ideally, this technique should be practiced for about 20 minutes during the day.

Another technique for deep sleep is abdominal breathing. By breathing from the abdomen and directing attention to the breath, relaxation can be achieved. Some people prefer lying down in a dimly lit room, listening to soft music, or closing their eyes while focusing on their breath. Placing hands on the belly and observing the gentle movement during inhalation and exhalation helps redirect the mind from busy thoughts to the body, facilitating a calm state conducive to sleep. This exercise can be practiced when lying down to fall asleep, as well as when waking up during the night and experiencing difficulty falling back asleep.

Affirmation meditation is similar to mindfulness meditation but involves replacing distractions that keep you awake with positive affirmations or mantras. By choosing an affirmation that resonates with you or using a mantra from a particular faith tradition, you can interrupt negative thought patterns and promote a calm state of mind. Positive bedtime affirmations are powerful tools for creating new neural pathways in the brain and strengthening beneficial beliefs while minimizing attention to stressors that hinder sleep.

Guided meditation is another technique that utilizes the soothing voice of a meditation teacher to help induce sleep. In a guided meditation session, an instructor provides guidance throughout the practice, instructing you to inhale deeply, exhale, and progressively relax different parts of your body. While having an instructor is not necessary, some individuals find it helpful. Imagining relaxing scenes, such as a beach or mountains, and engaging all the senses in the visualization can contribute to a calm state conducive to sleep.

Counting down is a technique where you imagine yourself descending stairs or a gentle hill while counting down from a chosen number. This exercise can be combined with abdominal breathing and progressive relaxation, further aiding relaxation and preparing the mind and body for sleep.

Gratitude meditation involves focusing on the things you are grateful for instead of the breath. This technique is simple yet effective for falling asleep, as there is always something to be grateful for, no matter how small or significant. By challenging yourself to think of the things you appreciate in life, you can shift your attention away from worries and induce

Chapter 20: Hypnosis Therapy for Sleep Improvement

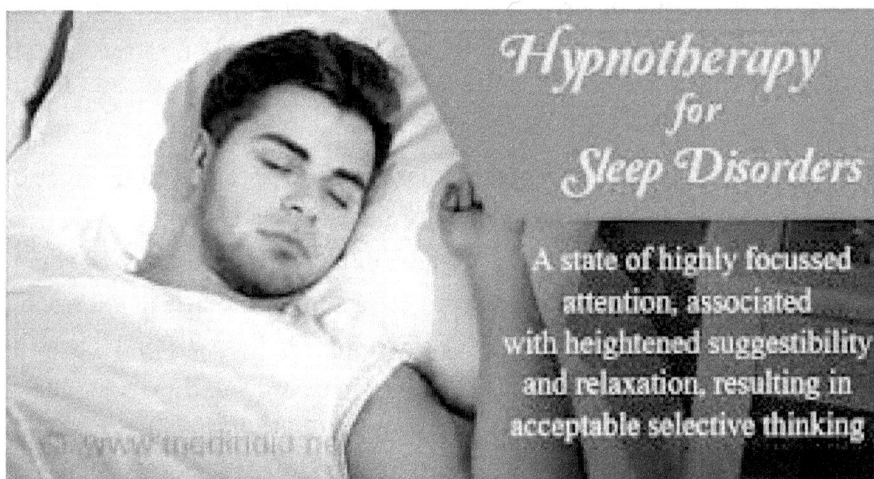

Self-hypnosis is a contemporary method that allows individuals to work with specially designed hypnosis audios to achieve their desired outcomes. It is crucial for patients to practice self-hypnosis in order to effectively incorporate hypnosis into therapy, including pain management during a trance state. The goal is to empower patients to utilize hypnosis independently, providing relief from pain whenever and wherever needed, regardless of their consultation circumstances.

Scientific research has demonstrated the efficacy of hypnosis in treating pain and various other conditions, making it a recognized therapeutic option in many countries' public healthcare systems. Prominent medical journals, such as Nature, Science, and Oncology, have published numerous studies supporting the use of hypnosis. Hospitals and clinics worldwide, including renowned institutions in Europe and the United States, utilize hypnosis in medical practice. It is utilized for pain management in specialized units, such as the Pain Unit of the Hospital Universitari de Tarragona in Spain and the Sleep Unit of the Madrid Rubber Clinic and La Pau Hospital in Madrid. Additionally, hypnosis is used in oncology as a complement to chemical anesthesia.

There are several misconceptions surrounding hypnosis that need clarification. Three common myths are as follows:

Aggravation of physical or mental illness: Hypnosis itself does not worsen physical or mental conditions, but the improper use of hypnosis during therapy can be harmful.

Control by the hypnotist: Hypnosis is a self-induced state, and the person undergoing hypnosis retains control. They have the ability to refuse suggestions that go against their morals or will, and they can terminate the hypnosis process whenever they wish.

Lack of effort from the patient: Although hypnosis can feel effortless and automatic during a session, the individual remains in an active state that requires effort. The patient's active participation and willingness are crucial for the effectiveness of hypnosis.

Quality sleep is essential for overall well-being, and hypnosis can be a valuable tool in achieving better sleep. If you have been struggling with sleep issues, sleep hypnosis can provide the relaxation and rest you need. While hypnosis is often known for its effectiveness in smoking cessation and overcoming phobias, its benefits for sleep improvement should not be overlooked.

Various factors can disrupt sleep, including stress, anxiety, changes in the sleeping environment, unhealthy eating habits, psychological disorders, and certain medications. Sleep hypnosis has been shown to promote deeper sleep, as evidenced by changes in brain wave activity, particularly an increase in slow-wave sleep, which is essential for physical and mental restoration. Deep sleep obtained through hypnosis can lead to fewer nocturnal awakenings, quicker sleep onset, and reduced pre-sleep worries.

Sleep hypnosis employs relaxation techniques and visualizations to induce healthy sleep patterns. With the guidance of a professional, muscle relaxation, controlled breathing, and the use of imagery can help individuals regain restful sleep. Sleep hypnosis also shields against external disturbances such as noise and stress, allowing for a peaceful sleep environment. Prioritizing quality sleep is crucial for restoring energy and maintaining overall well-being.

The consequences of inadequate sleep should not be underestimated. Sleep deprivation can lead to increased food consumption, weakened immune system, diminished physical attractiveness, decreased life expectancy, higher risk of accidents, and potential fertility issues. To address these concerns, sleep hypnosis aims to achieve goals such as physical and mental relaxation, visualization techniques, thought projection, learning to embrace sleep, and waking up feeling refreshed and content.

If you struggle with insomnia, hypnosis techniques can offer a viable solution. By specifically addressing the underlying causes of sleeplessness, such as stress and worries, hypnosis helps individuals disconnect from distractions and attain a state of relaxation conducive to sleep. Hypnosis audios designed for sleep and relaxation.

Chapter 21: Cultivating Inner Peace

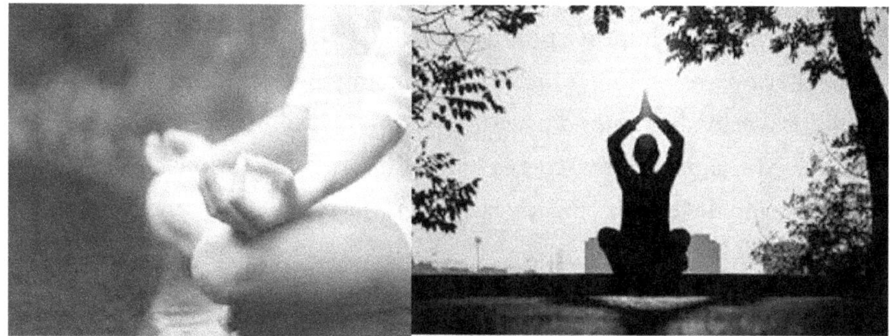

In this chapter, the author provides guidance on increasing inner peace through meditation. The first tip is to have a clear purpose and reason for meditating. Rather than solely aiming for general inner peace, it is suggested to focus on specific issues or goals, such as addressing stress or improving sleep. By identifying emotional and health needs, individuals can tailor their meditation practice accordingly.

The importance of being present in the moment is emphasized throughout the chapter. Developing the ability to quiet the mind and empty thoughts takes time and practice. By staying focused on short-term goals and practicing mindfulness, individuals can gradually work towards inner peace. Establishing a consistent time and place for meditation is recommended to create a ritual and form a healthy habit. Planning ahead helps eliminate distractions and promotes a stronger mind-body connection during meditation. It is acknowledged that interruptions may occur, and it is important to be kind to oneself and adapt to life's challenges.

The chapter concludes by introducing the benefits of meditation in various aspects of life. Mental health benefits are highlighted, including reducing depression and anxiety. Studies have shown that mindfulness meditation can be as effective as antidepressant drugs and can improve symptoms of depression. Performance benefits are also discussed, such as enhanced decision-making and improved focus and attention. Meditation is found to increase cognitive skills and may be beneficial for individuals with ADHD. Additionally, meditation can help relieve pain and has potential benefits for patients with conditions like fibromyalgia. By avoiding excessive multitasking, individuals can improve productivity and reduce stress. Physical benefits of meditation are explored, including reducing the risk of heart disease and stroke, lowering high blood pressure, and potentially promoting longevity. Lastly, meditation is presented as a tool for improving relationships, fostering empathy, and developing positive connections with oneself and others.

Chapter 22: Practicing Mindfulness

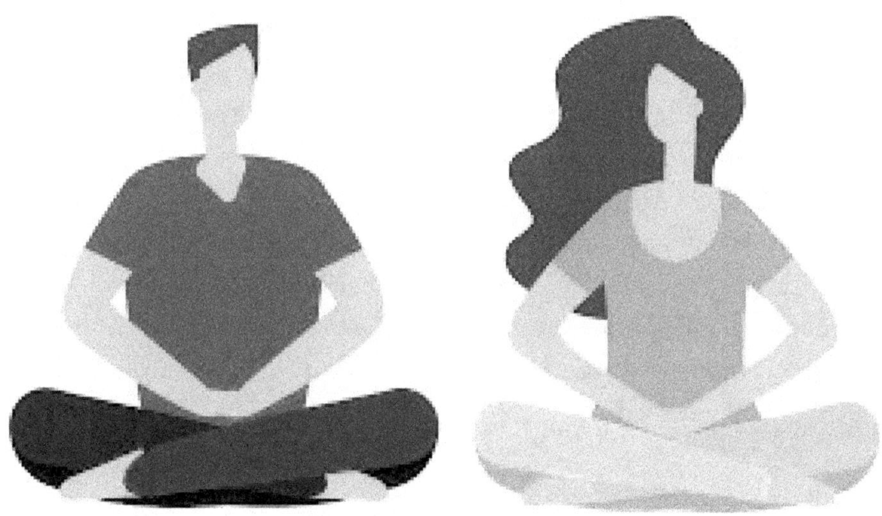

Mindfulness goes beyond formal meditation sessions. It can be practiced anywhere, not just when sitting with closed eyes and a straight back. To practice mindfulness, all you need is to be fully present in the moment without being carried away by thoughts or emotions. You don't require any special place or equipment; just make sure you won't be interrupted.

Learning this meditation technique is easy because it's straightforward. Simply find a quiet and comfortable space, free yourself from troubling thoughts, and engage in mindfulness meditation. You can incorporate mindfulness into various aspects of your life, such as when going to work, walking, practicing sports, or doing household activities.

There are no specific rules for mindfulness meditation. Any routine activity can be transformed into a mindfulness practice by bringing your full attention to it. Even washing dishes can be an opportunity for mindfulness meditation, as it provides a serene environment. By letting go and enjoying the experience, you can refresh your mind and find inner peace.

Another opportunity for meditation arises while brushing your teeth. Since it's a daily activity, there are no excuses not to meditate. Feel the brush in your hand, keep your feet firmly on the ground, and practice mindfulness meditation. You can also meditate while driving or during exercise, dedicating 10 minutes in the morning to mindfulness meditation.

The more you practice mindfulness, the easier it becomes to stay present and focused where you need to be, rather than being carried away by your wandering mind. The more you practice, the more you will benefit from it. The crucial thing is to start and work towards a regular practice of at least 15-20 minutes every day.

The Basics of Mindfulness Practice

In today's busy society, finding ten minutes for meditation may seem impossible due to our hectic schedules and essential responsibilities. Meditation is often seen as something limited to a specific group of people, particularly those who are depressed. However, once we realize the value of giving our minds some rest, we can create time to meditate. While we take care of our physical health, possessions, and appearance, we tend to neglect our minds, which shape our experience of life. Therefore, it's crucial to consider our minds as a precious possession and enhance their value through mindfulness.

Mindfulness can be practiced through formal meditation sessions or smaller moments throughout the day. To incorporate mindfulness into your day, follow these steps:

Set aside time for mindfulness meditation. You don't need any special equipment, but you do need to allocate a quiet space and time.

Observe the present moment as it is. The goal of mindfulness is simple: to become aware of the present moment without judgment.

Let judgments pass by. If any judgments arise during your mindfulness practice, simply notice them and let them go.

Bring your mind back to observing the present moment. Your mind may wander with thoughts from time to time, and that's normal. Be kind to yourself and gently redirect your attention back to the present moment.

Mindfulness is a simple concept, but it's not necessarily easy. The key is to keep practicing it regularly, and you will gradually see the benefits. Mindfulness practice helps us become aware of various aspects of life that impact our daily existence.

Techniques to Cultivate Mindfulness

Mindful Breathing

Mindful breathing is an excellent way to begin mindfulness practice as it helps quiet the mind and allows for a deeper experience of the present moment. Conscious breathing involves using the breath as an object of concentration, focusing solely on one breath instead of jumping between different thoughts or distractions

Conclusion

No more wasted evenings struggling with insomnia. No more frustration of being awake at odd hours in the morning. No more sacrificing sleep to insomnia. No more mornings ruined by stress, anxiety, and depression. Finally, you have discovered the solution to waking up relaxed and refreshed, fully restored after a good night's sleep. Hypnosis is the answer to your insomnia.

When it comes to hypnosis, many researchers focus on a sleep component known as "slow wave sleep," which is also referred to as deep sleep. Studies have found that hypnosis may increase the amount of time spent in slow wave sleep for individuals suffering from insomnia. This is promising news for those struggling with sleep deprivation.

By entering a state of slow wave sleep or deep sleep, you can allow your mind and body to fully relax and let go of the anxiety, stress, sadness, and pain caused by lack of sleep. Hypnosis can help you achieve this state of deep sleep, which is crucial for consolidating memories and healing your body and mind, leaving you feeling rejuvenated. Falling into a deep sleep is highly therapeutic, and another reason to consider hypnosis as a solution for your sleep problems.

Furthermore, research suggests that slow wave activity during the deep sleep stage is significantly enhanced following hypnosis. This indicates that hypnosis not only increases the duration of deep sleep but may also improve its quality. This could result in an easier time waking up in the morning, reduced stress and anxiety throughout the day, increased confidence, and decreased symptoms of depression.

Although hypnosis may not work for everyone, a key to successful hypnosis sessions is maintaining an open mind. When you approach guided hypnosis with an open mind, you become more suggestible. Increased suggestibility makes it easier for your mind to follow the prompts presented during the hypnosis session, leading to a successful session and ultimately successful sleep.

The connection between hypnosis and a good night's sleep is evident. If you have tried every solution available and still struggle to fall asleep, it can be incredibly frustrating. Tossing and turning every night leaves you exhausted and irritable, significantly impacting your quality of life. But now, there is another solution for you. Hypnosis can guide you towards a more fulfilling sleep, not only helping you fall asleep faster but also improving the quality of your sleep. Many other solutions may have fallen short, but now you have the secret to achieving restful sleep. The hypnosis sessions can be used as often as you need them, serving as a tool to sleep your way into the life you want to lead: a life of happiness and relaxation. You have explored the benefits of sleep hypnosis and its potential as a solution for insomnia. You have experienced its effectiveness through these four highly successful guided meditations. You are ready to enhance your quality of life by improving your sleep. Sleep well.

* 9 7 8 3 9 8 8 3 1 5 6 1 8 *